21 Day Sugar Detox: A Step By Step Guide For Beginners

GET ENERGIZED AND LOSE FAT BY BEATING THE SUGAR ADDICTION

Disclaimer

What You Will Find In This eBook?

Is your blood sugar out of balance?

Is your sweet tooth getting the best of you?

The *21 Day Sugar Detox: A Step By Step Guide For Beginners* contains the following:

1. Why the 21 day sugar detox works for you.
2. The importance of balanced blood sugar.
3. Step by step guide to carry out the detox plan.
4. What foods to eat and what to avoid.
5. A supportive walk through when you are going through this cleanse.
6. The psychology of curbing the cravings.
7. Meal plans.

So go ahead and try out the three week detox and experience what it feels like to break the hearts of many sugar-laden-food selling establishments!

Contents

Disclaimer 2

What You Will Find In This eBook? 3

You Know It When You Know It 8

What Is a Detox? 9

Why Is Sugar Bad For You? 10

    An Empty Calorie 10

    When Your Stomach Suddenly Decides To Imitate a Bottomless Pit 11

    The Ugly Duckling 12

    Dental Decay 13

    Gives You Diabetes 14

    Makes You Fat 15

    The Sweet Devil 16

Why is Sugar Hell Bent On Imitating Drugs? 17

    The Science of Why Sugar Cravings Are Annoying 19

    Where is sugar likely hidden? 20

    The Many Names Of Sugar 21

    What Causes The High Rush and The Sudden Low Feeling We Get When We Consume Sugar? 22

The Steps to Get You Started On The 21 Day Sugar Detox 23

    The Positive Symptoms During The 21 Day Cleanse 25

    The Negative symptoms that people report during The 21 day regime 26

The Amazing Benefits of Sugar Detox 27

Meal Plan Examples - To Get You Started 28

    Day 1 28

    Day 2 29

Detox Beverages 30

The Must Know Facts about The 21 Day Sugar Detox 32

    The Glycemic Index 32

    Fructose 33

    Carbs and Starch 34

    Protein 35

    Water 36

    Clean Your Diet 37

Lemon to The Rescue 38

Squats, Squats, Squats! 39

The Psychological Effects: How To Best Cope With What You Might Be Feeling......... 40

What Does Sugar Mean To Me? 41

What You Can Do: 42

   1.   Be Patient; Be Committed... 42

   2.   The Written Game Plan.. 43

   3.   Fill In The Spaces 44

   4.   Buddy Up 45

   5.   Let the World Know.. 46

   6.   Spring Clean the Kitchen 47

   7.   Meditation Helps 48

   8.   The Heart Wants What It Wants... 49

   9.   One Thought at A Time 50

The Perfect Escape Plan

Most of us think we did not consume any sugar each day unless we go on an eating spree that has our mouth lined with chocolate syrup and powdered sugar coating the corners. Not a pretty picture, right?

The fact is that all the processed foods that have dominated our lives are involuntarily stuffing our stomachs' with unhealthy sugar and carbs.

It is incredibly difficult to switch or let go of an entire chunk that makes up your lifestyle, especially since we grew up to find solace in sugary snacks. In eighth grade they had nice manners and never dared to make us fat! They were quiet companions and did not pass judgment on our choice of late night chick flicks and they were there in college when Romeo made a run for it.

So you wake up one day and witness the scale tipping, wondering how you can learn to tip the scales in your favor (tip: the figures never change). Let me break it down for you: the 21 Day Sugar Detox method is not a scam.

I use the word 'method', because unlike other weight loss and health enhancing practices, this is not a lifestyle change. It is more of a cleanse.

First off, the thing that most of us need to learn is that the _amount_ of food you consume does not lead to the atrocities of weight gain. It is the _type_ of food your body is taking in that determines whether you have enough to counter the bad effects of a cheat meal you had. The thing worth crying out in happiness about this detox is that it does not involve starving yourself or limiting yourself to liquid foods like most cleansing methods do (Hats off to Diane Sanflippo, savior of the female race).

Let's face it, we are a bunch of sugar rushed people afraid of dealing with the withdrawal that depriving ourselves of these treats will result in. It is high time that we paved our way out of the mess of imbalanced diets and sugar levels and treat ourselves to some good and healthy nutrition. After all, it is only a matter of 21 days.

You Know It When You Know It

The 21 Day Sugar Detox is most recommended when your blood sugar is hovering out of the bounds of control. How on Earth do you know it's the blood sugar and not bipolar disorder? Simple! Thankfully (or not) the blood sugar when out of balance sprouts some symptoms that you might notice.

1. If you feel some sort of fatigue after you are done with a meal, it could mean that either your blood sugar is too low or too high.
2. When you experience light headedness after missing out or skipping meals on purpose.
3. When you experience untimely cravings for food products like bread, lone sugar and sweets this is a definite sign of your blood sugar demanding attention.
4. When you do not feel the satisfaction you expect after curbing your craving for something sugary.
5. When you are going through life depending on caffeine to function properly at work or just to start off the day.
6. When you have tried numerous different ways to honestly lose weight and you are having trouble while others who started out with you are not.

Setting your blood sugar back into balance is not something new. Conventionally, people just sat back consumed more protein and fiber or reduced their intake of sources rich in simple carbohydrates and sugar.

The problem is that unfortunately today our daily lives are dominated by processed food so much that we almost feel bad to say no to such close affiliates in or lives; as opposed to the organic stuff our ancestors ate.

What Is a Detox?

The term detox can mean several different things to different people. Some resort to this for weight loss others for cleansing the body or simply fasting. The word detox simply denotes the activity of ridding the human body of toxic or harmful substances. You might be thinking that it's one of the body's functions to naturally cleanse all toxic and harmful matter. The fact is that our body gets overwhelmed by the traffic of all the unhealthy food we are consuming that it falls under serious need for a helping hand. Today we are exposed to more toxins and pollutants than ever before.

What is more important is that we make long term permanent changes in our lifestyle and diet but detoxing does the trick to support our natural cleansing system by sharing its load for a while.

Why Is Sugar Bad For You?

Knowing why sugar is to blame for all the bad things happening in your life right now is a great way to motivate yourself to take the sugar free detox journey.

An Empty Calorie

Did you know that sugar has zero nutritional value? The victual is literally dubbed "the anti-nutrient". When we consume sugar our digestive tract has to make use of energy deposits just to process the glucose molecules.

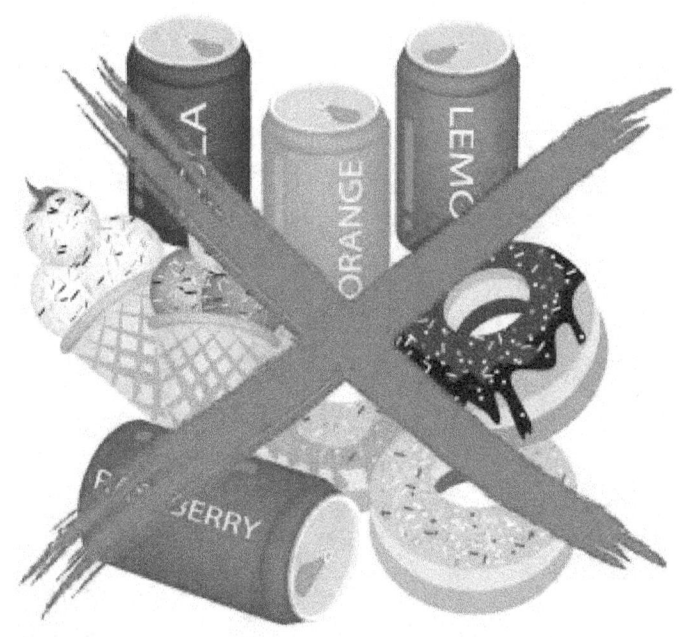

When Your Stomach Suddenly Decides To Imitate a Bottomless Pit

The other problem with sugar is that if you eat food rich in sugar, your digestive tract starts digesting the calories but it never comes across any nutrients so no matter how much sugar you eat, your body will send you signals of unfulfilled feelings; that's the blood stream crying out for some nutrition! This is essentially why foods rich in protein and veggies are a great source of nutrition and automatically have you feeling full after you are done with them.

And now we know why women avoid them. Psychologically it might seem like you had something fatty and ate too much. Well trust me, in the 21 Day Detox plan you will need this to function!

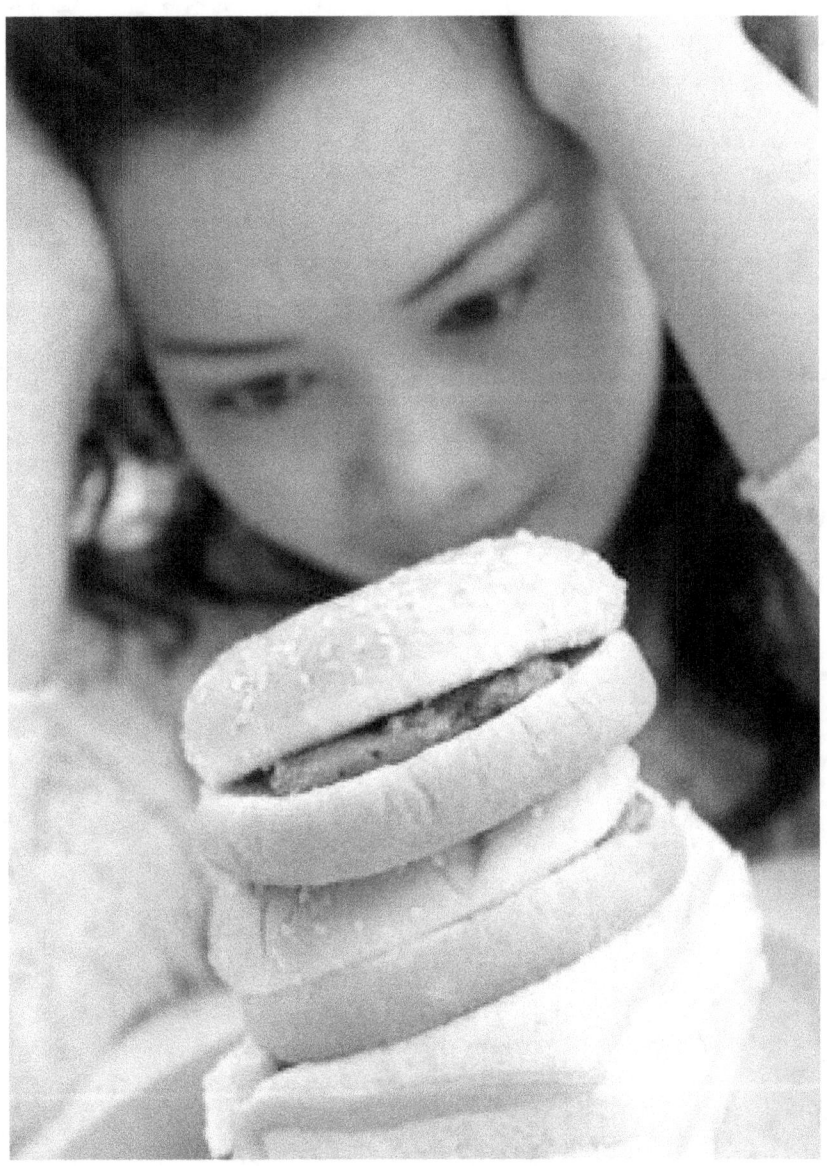

The Ugly Duckling

Sugar causes the ugly duckling effect in reverse. From a swan you are reduced to a helpless duckling. Facts are that sugar causes many skin problems like acne, dark and puffy circles under the eyes and can make the skin look oily. Moreover it is the refined sugar that we eat that lowers the creation of collagen molecules in our body. Collagen is a protein that is essential in making the skin look naturally young and keeps it tight. To add to this, sugar is also the culprit to all those insomnia ridden nights you have had. Too much sugar robs you of your quality sleep. Moving on to the list of bad skin care effects, refined sugar also cuts down on the quantity of Vitamin B in your body. These vitamins are important for a healthy nervous system, nails, hair and several other organs in the body.

Just imagine the colossal damage that you will be avoiding by cutting sugar out of your life.

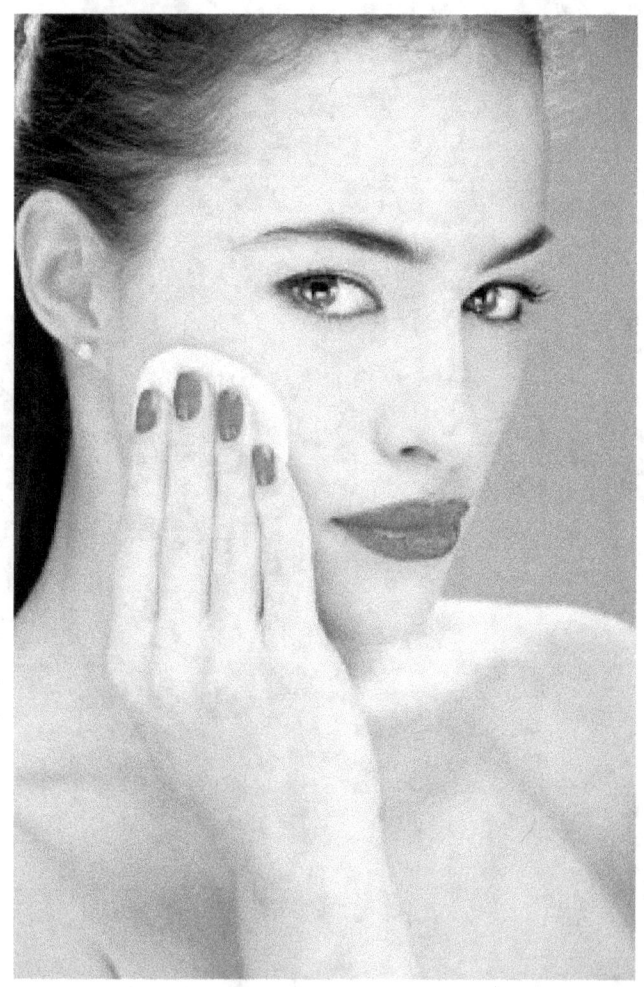

Dental Decay

Let's not get carried away beyond the obvious. Think about it, would you not do anything for the perfect set of flashy teeth? What we were taught as kids was not only limited to implementing in a young age. Sugar leads to dental decay by producing and enhancing bacterial growth in the mouth, it changes the pH and is the reason why there is that stubborn white cover on your tongue. Eating excessive sugar leads to diseases like paradentosis.

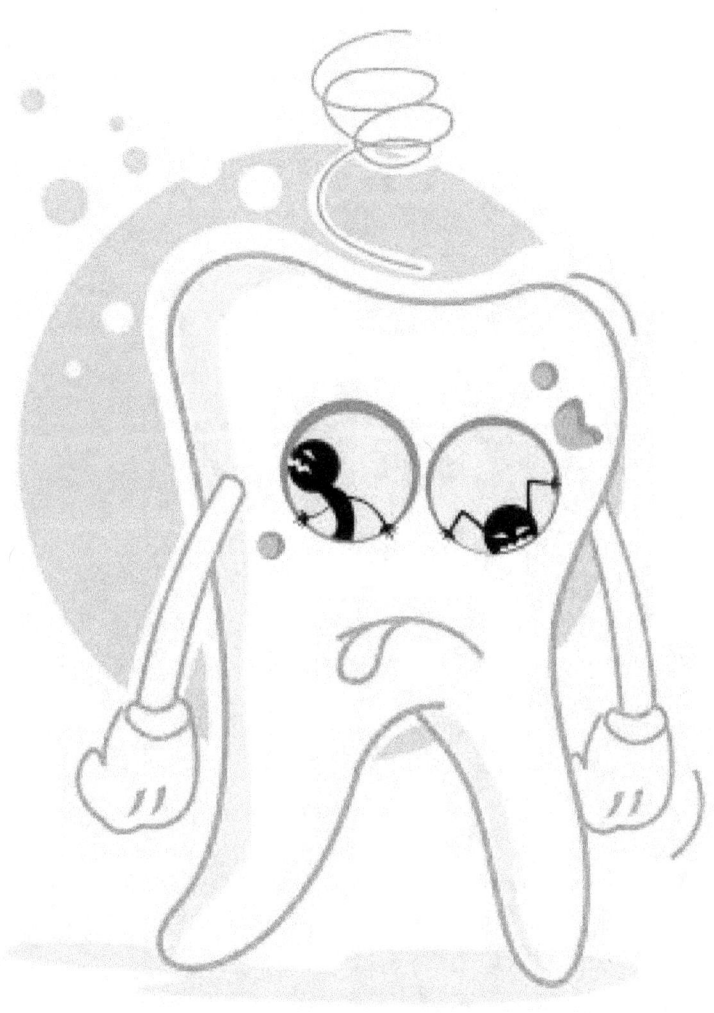

Gives You Diabetes

Diabetes mellitus type II is caused solely by excessive consumption of sugar. Today the stats for this disease are rocketing as compared to the years before. It is fast becoming common in teenagers and young children. For instance having a can of soft drink does not mean you had very minimal sugar. Do the math! You actually consumed 150 calories and 10 whole spoonfuls of sugar in ten minutes.

What happens is that too much sugar in the human body boosts the levels of triglycerides. This is the circulation of the fat in your body. This is how sugar is indirectly connected to heart diseases and the rising cholesterol levels. Get rid of sugar if you don't like the idea of heart attacks.

Makes You Fat

A bit of sugar consumption is not directly proportional to the weight you gain. When you eat sugar your body turns the simple carbs into glucose in the blood stream. It takes a lot of heavy and intense exercise to reduce this glucose from the blood stream. If it is not done, then the organ, the pancreas, if forced to keep releasing insulin which makes the cells in your body sponge up all the excess glucose and store it as fat. This ultimately makes you fat and heavy on the bathroom scale.

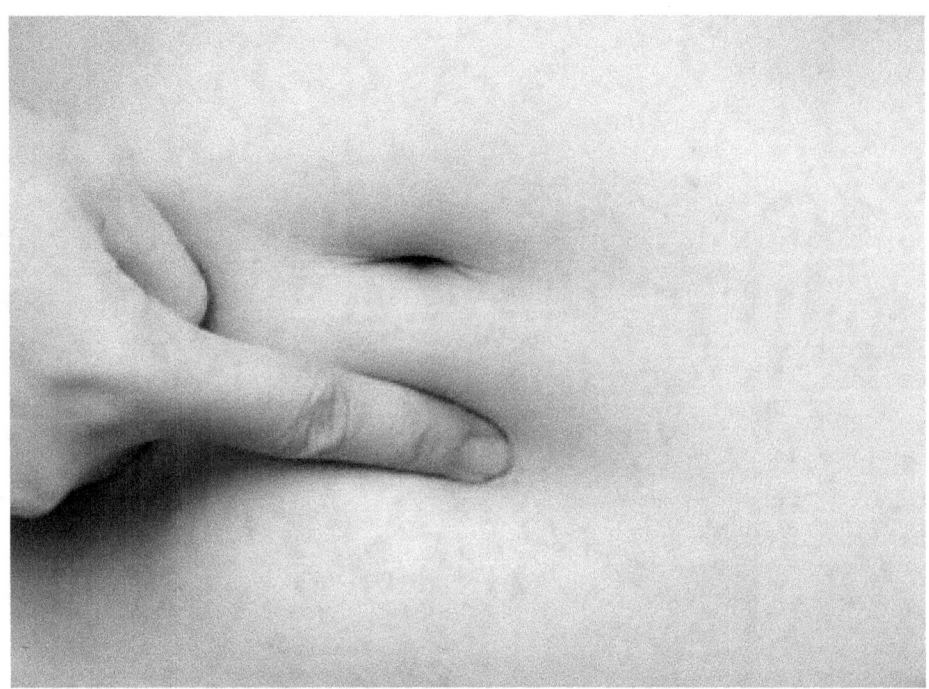

The Sweet Devil

Sugar however tempting it may be causes a lot of other unwanted and unhealthy effects to the human body. In the stomach with the aid of specific bacteria and yeast it creates alcohol fermentation, in this same way it also encourages the growth of pathogenic bacteria. This allows unhealthy blood to flow to the liver which in turn makes the liver unhealthy and with the disturbed functioning of the liver, unhealthy blood is sent to the rest of the body, organs, and cells too.

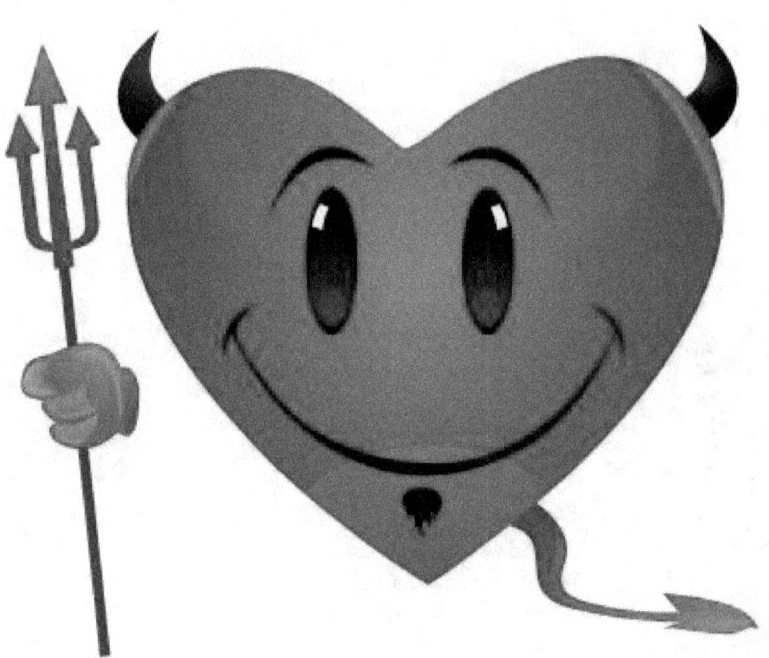

Why is Sugar Hell Bent On Imitating Drugs?

Ever thought through the idea of letting go of sugar? When did it become the enemy and what is wrong with the world? At first everyone had a problem with fat and now suddenly we are taught to hate sugar? Something must not be right.

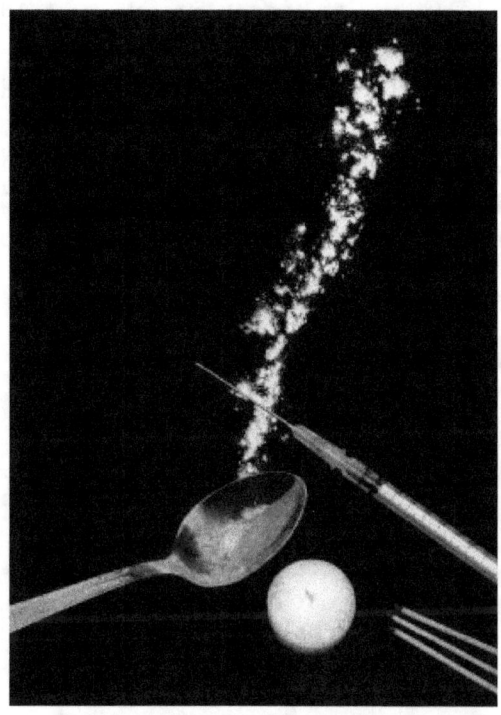

Well it is high time that we believe that something is. Let's be honest and rational. The world is fighting increased levels of obesity and cardiac diseases. Sugar has been linked with diseases like diabetes, premature aging, specific cancers and kidney illnesses.

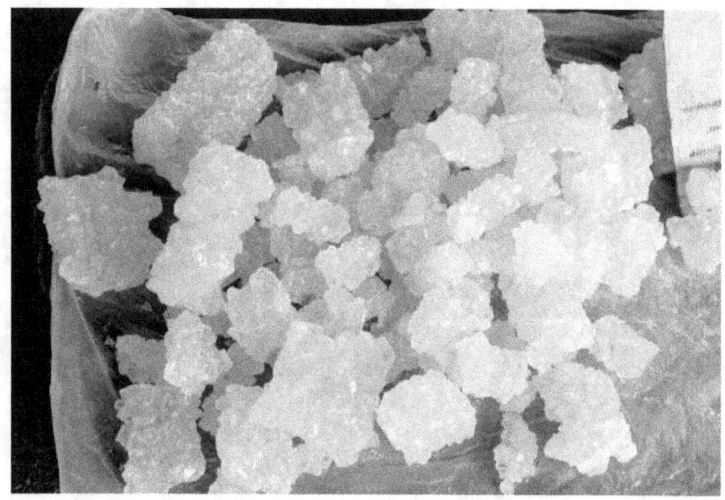

The bad news is that sugar today has learned the art of stealth and is hidden in every other thing that you find for yourself. It is everywhere, in the fiber stripped rice, tinned veggies, etc. Let's not blame the manufacturers… just yet.

By incorporating sugar in processed food that moves off the shelf each day they could control the quantity of processed victuals we buy by overriding our sensors with more sugar so that our demanding desire matches it every time we are purchasing that product again… now you may blame them whole heartedly. Think about it, when your mother says the sauce has changed over the decades, it is not because you purchased the wrong tin it is because over the years the sugar quantity has accumulated considerably.

The Science of Why Sugar Cravings Are Annoying

So how exactly does nutritionist class sugar addiction compare next to the Class A drug cocaine? This theory was tested in France in 2009. The study was done on rodents that were already addicted to cocaine. It harvested the results that showed that the rats opted for sugar around 8 times more than they chose cocaine.

So what in reality happens when you have sugar? When you consume sugar, chemicals in your body that make feelings of euphoria are released (opioids) and dopamine which helps to control the brains pleasure and reward center is triggered. This means that when the sugar you eat hits the brain your sensors that indicate pain are turned off. This happy indicator makes you want to have sugar again and again to ward off any unhappy feeling.

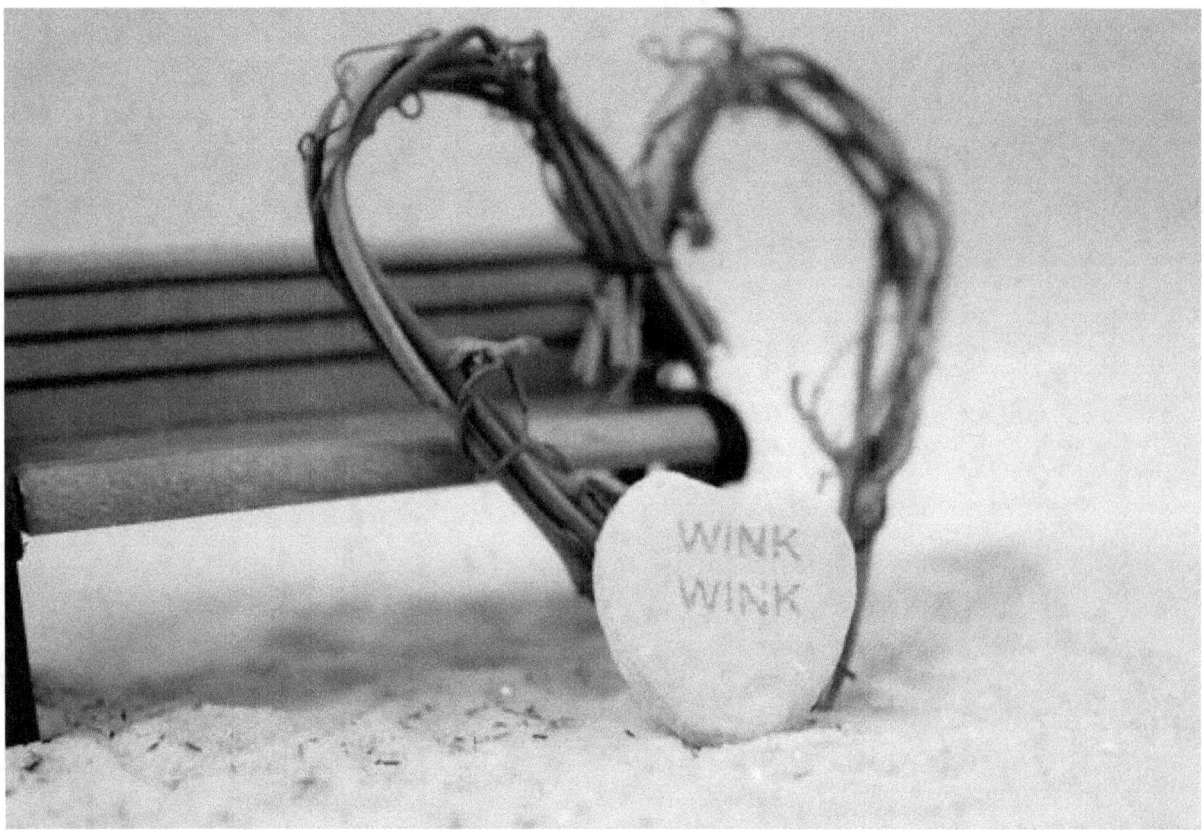

Since sugar has been evidently categorized as an addictive substance and like all addictive elements it is desired more and more as you consume it. This is due to the fact that anything we have too much dulls our taste bud to the taste of them and thus we want more and more of that food to feel the same sugary taste on our tongue.

Where is sugar likely hidden?

Now you must remember that here we are mainly concerned about the sugar that is hidden and we consume these foods without realizing our sugar intake. Sugar is hidden in packaged foods. When we eliminate the use of pre-processed foods just because we are laying off sugar we are doing ourselves the favor of eradicating many other chemicals and preservatives that we might have also unknowingly consumed.

Fruits on the other hand are organic and healthy, but during your sugar detox you cannot have too many as it too can cause high sugar levels in your blood.

Maintaining even blood sugar is the basic factor to weight loss. Even if you take up the detox to balance the uneven sugar levels in your blood stream, losing weight and excessive fat from your body is just another bonus.

The Many Names Of Sugar

High fructose corn syrup, fructose and rice syrup are all sugars. Other forms are artificial sweeteners even though their main aim is to counteract the bad effects of sugar unfortunately it fails on that front so it is best not to ever go for these. If you are wondering how a widely used product could not come to terms here is why: Artificial sweeteners do not contain calories but they do however work effectively to make the human body think that it consumed its quota of sugar. This is not as good a thing as it sounds because making the body think that it had sugar by the use of a placebo does not prevent it from the reaction which is that the body starts releasing insulin. These extra insulin levels are torture on your sugar cravings and make you feel like you should have more sugar.

So the bottom line is that if you want to curb your sugar cravings then don't have sugar or the artificial kind either. Face the cravings dead in the eye. You will scare them away for sure. The secret is: Do Not Give Up!

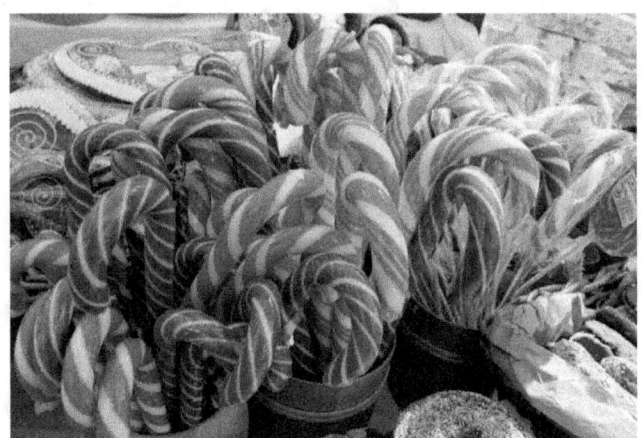

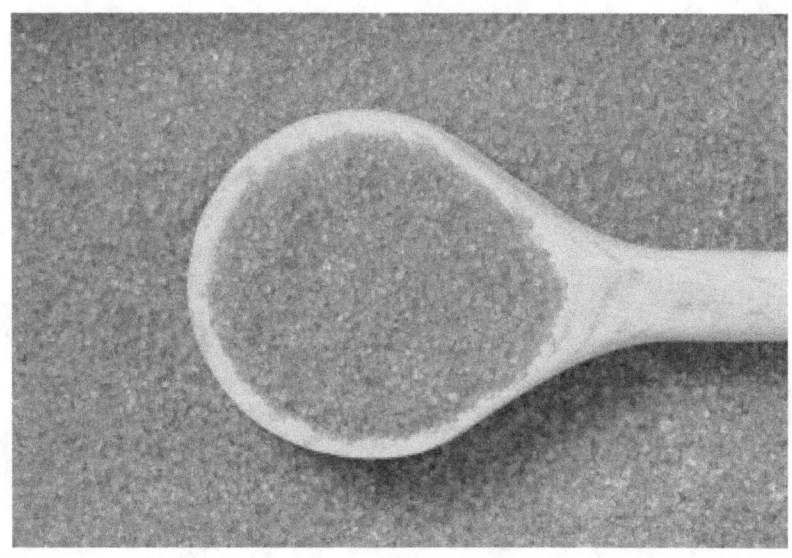

What Causes The High Rush and The Sudden Low Feeling We Get When We Consume Sugar?

When we eat foods that spike our sugar level, we crash, get tired and eat something to balance it out. The sugar detox is meant to prevent this; you will need to eat when you feel hungry though it's hardly likely that you will.

The Steps to Get You Started On The 21 Day Sugar Detox

This is pretty simple. The first step is to mentally mark out all the food items you eat that have sugar and carbs in them and then make a promise to file a restraining order against them.

Next refer to the food list that will follow in the next pages and eat the ones that are recommended and good for you.

Now the most important part about this is that if you get tempted and give in to eat the foods you should avoid you must start the 21 day regime from day one all over again.

What You Might Experience During Your three Weeks Of Detoxing

At first when you suddenly let go of your daily and normal intake of sugar your body will cry out in the form of more pronounced sugar cravings. After 3 days these awful cravings will learn to ease down and you will experience zero cravings all of a sudden. Remember the first couple of days require the most will power because as time goes on it is easier for you to keep off the sugar. So don't give in the first few days.

Now when the cravings stop your energy levels will automatically boost up and this is the point when you might feel as if it is okay to have a piece of flour bread or eat moderate amounts of food. At this time you must remember that the 21 Day Detox is a cleanse and not a lifestyle so what you want to enjoy will come but **after** the 21 days. When your cravings stop you may also feel a difference in your skin which is a great way to motivate yourself to keep the diet up.

You would feel much better and will keep up the detox if you face the facts. Remember it is the sugar in your diet that makes you obese and your skin dull and ugly, not the fat. One of the properties of sugar is to target and deteriorate the collagen in your skin. Also consuming carbs and sugar together is the main reason why people are tired all the time.

In America the stats say that on average a person eats 3 pounds of sugar each week and that is not from sweets alone. The thing is that all the processed foods that dominate our lives have too much sugar in them and we do not even realize this. This leads to our body releasing insulin and this insulin level leads to excessive weight gain.

Any sugarholic will tell you how difficult it is to get off sugar. Some recovering sugarholics will start by eradicating small amounts of sugar from their diet in hopes that one day it will be all gone but it does not work that way. Sugar is difficult to get off just like cocaine and in order to get off the victual completely you must limit yourself to strict and zero intake of the food.

The Positive Symptoms During The 21 Day Cleanse

During the cleanse you will experience definite fat loss, you will sleep better at night, your body will show lower cholesterol levels, your mood will brighten considerably and this may break into a habit. This means very low chances for depression. You will experience increased levels of energy and more consistent energy too; your metabolism will improve, you will feel your palate adjusting to the healthy foods, you will notice how clear your skin has become, you won't only experience fat loss but less bloating too and of course your sugar cravings will be eliminated too.

The Negative symptoms that people report during The 21 day regime

These effects only occur the first few days and then are no longer present. First off as a supposed sugarholic this sudden withdrawal of sugar from your body will leave you more emotionally sensitive. You might experience headaches (don't worry it's not caused by anything serious just the cravings), you might feel irritable all the time, have rashes or your skin breaking out in some way due to this sudden change in your diet, also some people report to have bad breath but it still cannot be proved whether it is because of the detox, mucus drainage, mind constantly wandering to old memories, sporadic sleep, body odor, gas, constipation, feelings of lethargy and reduced energy.

So It's Perfectly Easy You Say

All the negative effects that one might experience in the very first couple of days may not be experienced by everyone, and not all of them coupled together either. Now the good news is that these symptoms are also an indicator that the detox is working. What some might call the "healing crisis" during a cleanse. Basically what your body is doing is that it is working to clean everything from the inside, and that too is at a fast pace. But you must remember everyone reacts to a cleanse differently.

Eyes On The Prize

The positive things that you are rewarded after the cleanse are:

Significant fat loss, which means considerable weight loss.

1. You will notice how your skin condition has improved.
2. You will sleep better.
3. Your cholesterol will be under control.
4. Your mood will spike in positivity.

The Amazing Benefits of Sugar Detox

It is literally beyond any one's capability to list all the benefits that you get to reap after the successful implementation of the 21 Day Sugar Detox.

Well first off the best thing about the sugar detox is that it functions effectively to get rid of all the fat and toxins in your diet without you having to starve yourself or be restricted to a diet plan that excludes so many everyday foods.

Now the only thing in the diet that you are not consuming is the sugary foods and snacks. But guess what? The 21 Day Sugar Detox comes with an array of substitute foods so it literally becomes difficult to say that you are really on any sort of hard diet. This design was created so that the 21 Day Sugar Detox does not suffer from the same failure rate many other diets have. No one wants to give up in the middle of any diet or cleanse regime. It all makes the entire practice a waste of time.

After the program many people report that they feel much better than they ever had in years. Others reported that they had a more positive outlook towards everything which also strangely led them to perform better at everything.

Meal Plan Examples - To Get You Started

Day 1

For Breakfast:

½ cup scrambled egg whites; 1 cup baby spinach leaves; tomatoes and bell pepper.

For Lunch:

1 cup Pasta Tuna Salad cooked whole grain with 1 cup chopped cherry tomatoes; water packed tuna salad with 2 chopped onions, 2 teaspoons olive oil and 1 teaspoon vinegar dressing.

For Snack:

Avocado smoothie with spinach, ginger, cinnamon and green tea.

For Dinner:

2 cups field greens cooked in 2 teaspoons olive oil; 1 sweet potato (boiled); 5 Oz grilled chicken breast.

Day 2

For Breakfast:

1 cup oatmeal, ¼ cup Greek yogurt and 1 banana, 1 apple and 5 grapes.

For Lunch:

Salad: Small spinach leaves, pinch of salt, 1 teaspoon vinegar dressing, 2 teaspoons olive oil, 1 avocado, ¼ cup chickpeas, ½ cup quinoa and red and green bell peppers. Add in a cup of cucumber slices.

For Snack:

Green Tea

For Dinner:

1 cup lemon water, cucumber and mint; 1 cup broccoli and winter squash; ¼ cup brown rice (cook these in ½ Oz olive oil so they will become ½ cup brown rice); 1 salmon filet.

Detox Beverages

Fruit juices have huge quantities of sugar. They are no doubt refreshing and healthy. For instance, 9 Oz orange juice has 10.5 grams of sugar. The same quantity of Coca Cola has 26 grams of sugar.

The average human body is made up of 70 % water. This water that we have consumed needs to be replaced as soon as it reaches the bladder. If we do not flush our systems it is going to get old very fast. The bigger your body is the more water you need. On average a healthy body needs 2 to 3 liters of water.

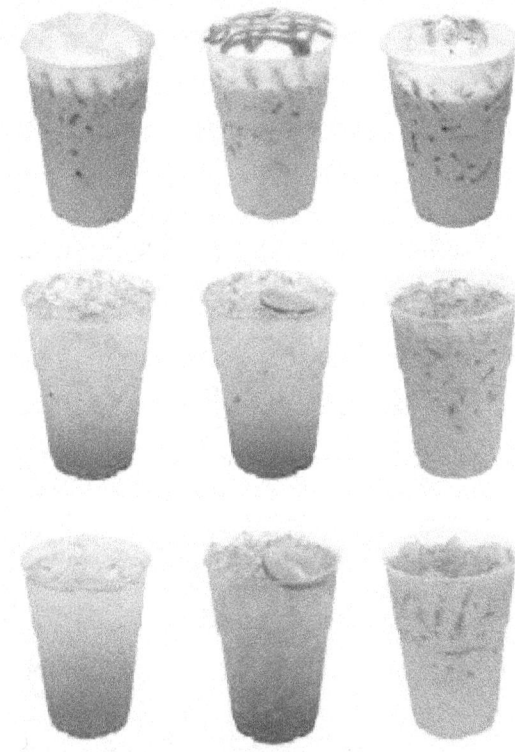

Now to stop yourself from regular water breaks add some mineral salts to the water like sodium bicarbonate. This will also keep the pH and electrolyte balance stable.

Though the sugar detox is not directly linked to caffeine. Beverages like coffee and tea are usually not recommended. So it is best if you avoid them if you are not addicted. Studies show that caffeine is great for exercise and performance. Looking at black teas and coffee from a health perspective the caffeine lowers the red blood cells' efficiency and this leads to it lowering the flow of oxygen around the red blood cells.

The Must Know Facts about The 21 Day Sugar Detox

The best part about the sugar detox is that after you are successful with the 21 days of abstinence a little amount of sugar will feel way too sweet to you. Do not call the detox a diet plan; lets refer it as a health plan because that is all it is offering.

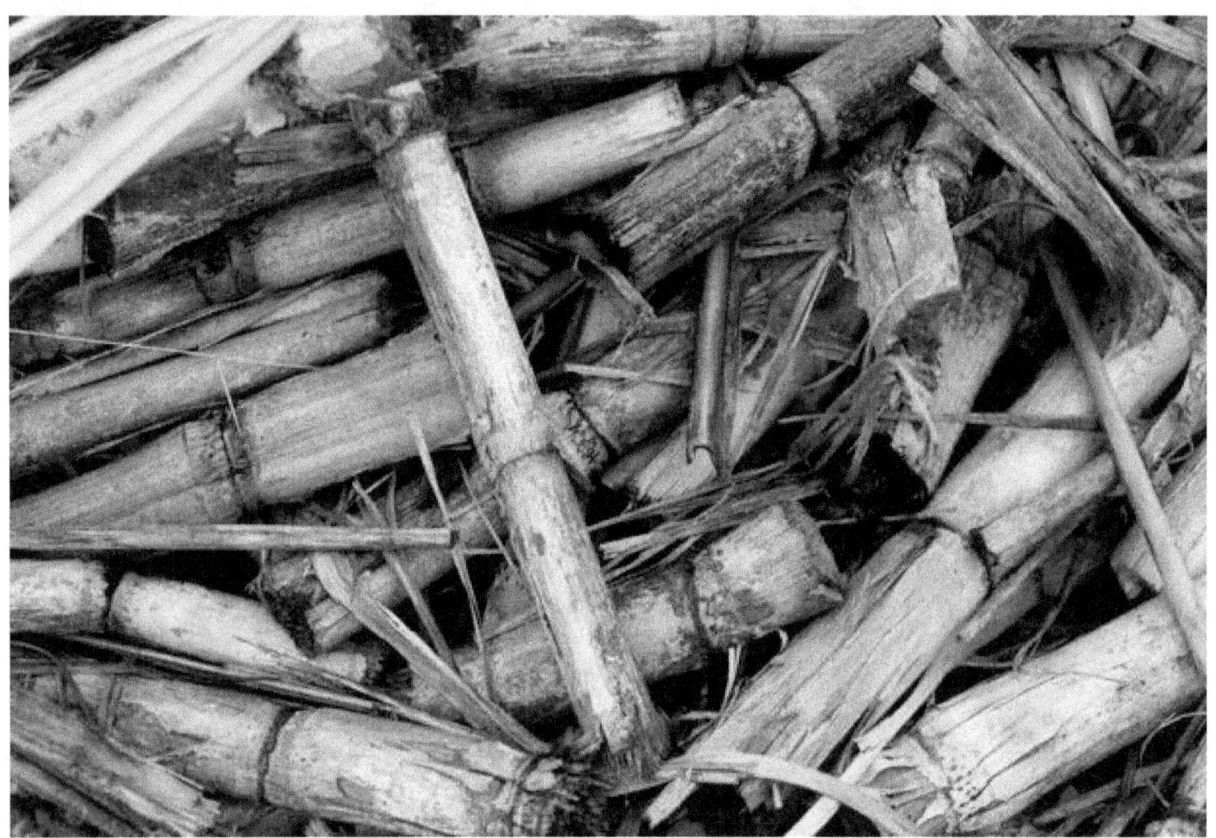

The Glycemic Index

The food detox revolves around this. Your glycemic index measures by the amount your blood sugar rises after you consume specific foods. The idea is to keep it as low as possible so that blood sugar levels are always balanced. So you need foods that are low in this during your 21 day sugar detox session.

Fructose

Next up you need to be super careful about the fructose levels in your diet too. Fructose is a simple sugar form found in honey, fruits and even vegetables so you must be careful around that front too. If you must have fructose it should be well under the limit of 20 g per day.

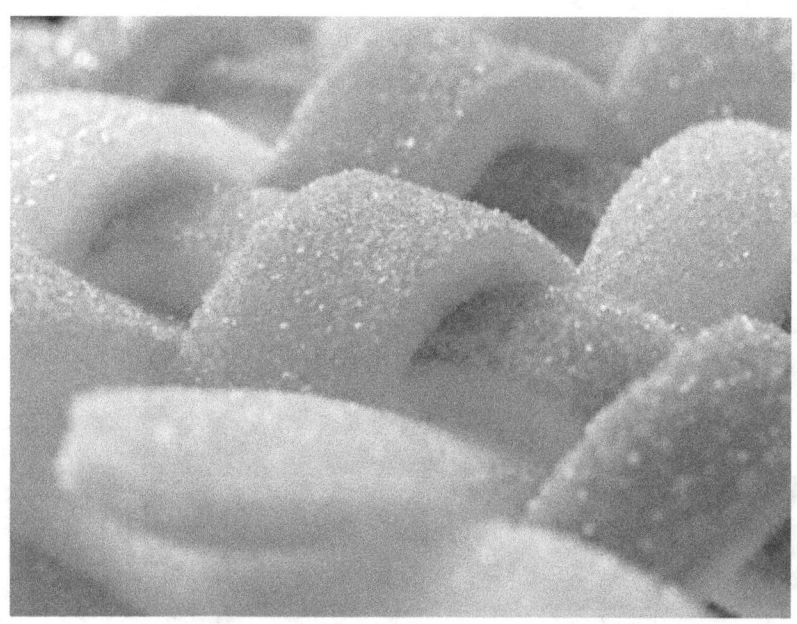

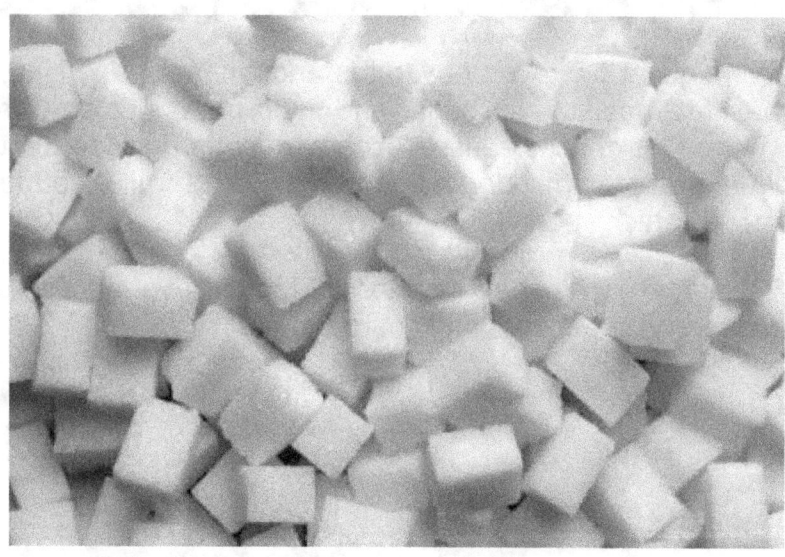

Carbs and Starch

A sugar detox also encourages that you do not consume carbs. This means that starchy foods are not to be eaten like bread, rice and pasta which people have almost every day. But you can however intake vegetable carbohydrates that help you lower your blood sugar.

Cheese, milk and yogurt is what you should be avoiding in your first three days of the detox. This kick starts an accelerated cleanse and prepares your body for the next days to come.

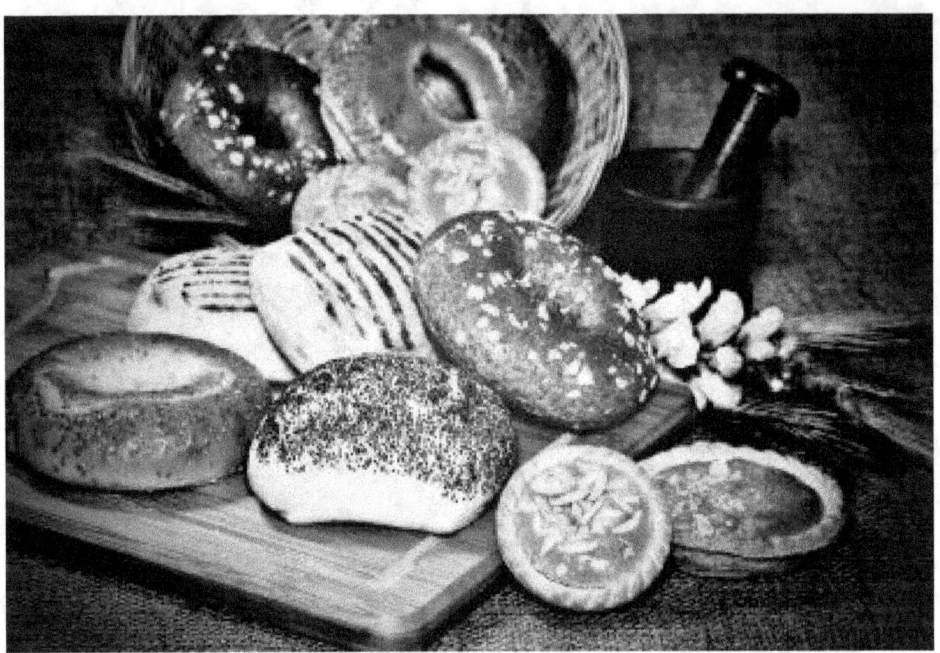

You cannot have carbohydrates and wheat of any kind. Artificial sweeteners are not a healthy substitute for sugar and must not under any circumstances be incorporated in your sugar detox cleanse. Alcohol must be avoided throughout the cleanse. Lemon and lime are recommended as good sources of fruit if you feel you need some in your daily menu, which you will.

To fill the gap that all the starchy foods have left out; good choices would be to have mushrooms, peppers and courgettes.

Protein

Now the things that you can learn to love and live with for a continuous 21 days are rich protein sources like eggs, fish and lean meat. Certain veggies are a good source of protein too like beans, chickpeas and lentils.

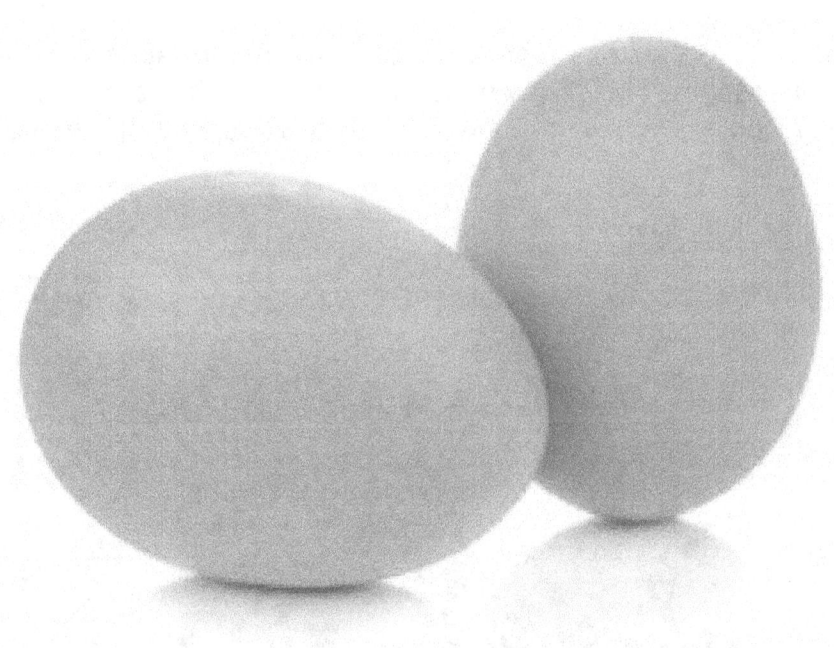

Water

A great component of your daily intake must be H$_2$O. Herbal teas aside, it is very essential that you drink lots and lots of water each day. Every day your daily intake of water must be more than 2 liters. The detox does allow a cup of unsweetened black coffee each day if you keep up the rest of your diet especially when it comes to hydration.

When you are up for cooking, remember nothing is better than olive oil or better yet coconut oil for cooking your food. Plus if you cannot figure out how to liven up your food simply use various herbs and spices. Your food will taste great, people will beg you for recipes, no harm will be done to the detox and all will be well with the world.

I understand that the sugar detox repeatedly screams out the tagline of "losing weight" but remember a cleanse like the 21 day sugar detox is not suitable at all for people who work out intensively, unless you want to black out in the middle of the exercise then it is great!

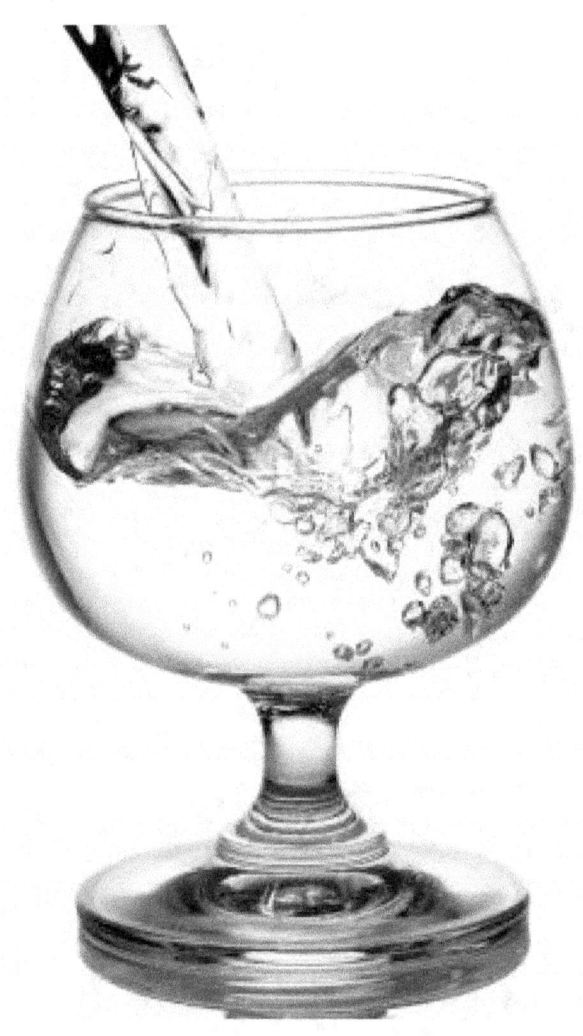

Clean Your Diet

Here is another neat trick that will help you easily get through the 21 days of detox: eat clean meals. This means that you need to avoid pre-cooked food as much as you can. Avoid having soybean oil and corn oil in your diet as these are hydrogenated oils. Foods like margarine can also come under this category as it is deformed from its natural state and then packaged.

A lot of people take supplements like Chromium per day to curb the cravings. However, I do not recommend this. There is no safer and natural way to curb the cravings other than enduring it for a few days on those afternoons that you are so used to partnering up with sugar. Find a new companion instead.

Lemon to The Rescue

Adding only 4 tablespoons of lemon juice to your diet will reduce the blood sugar impact in your blood stream. It's best if you consume it before you have a meal.

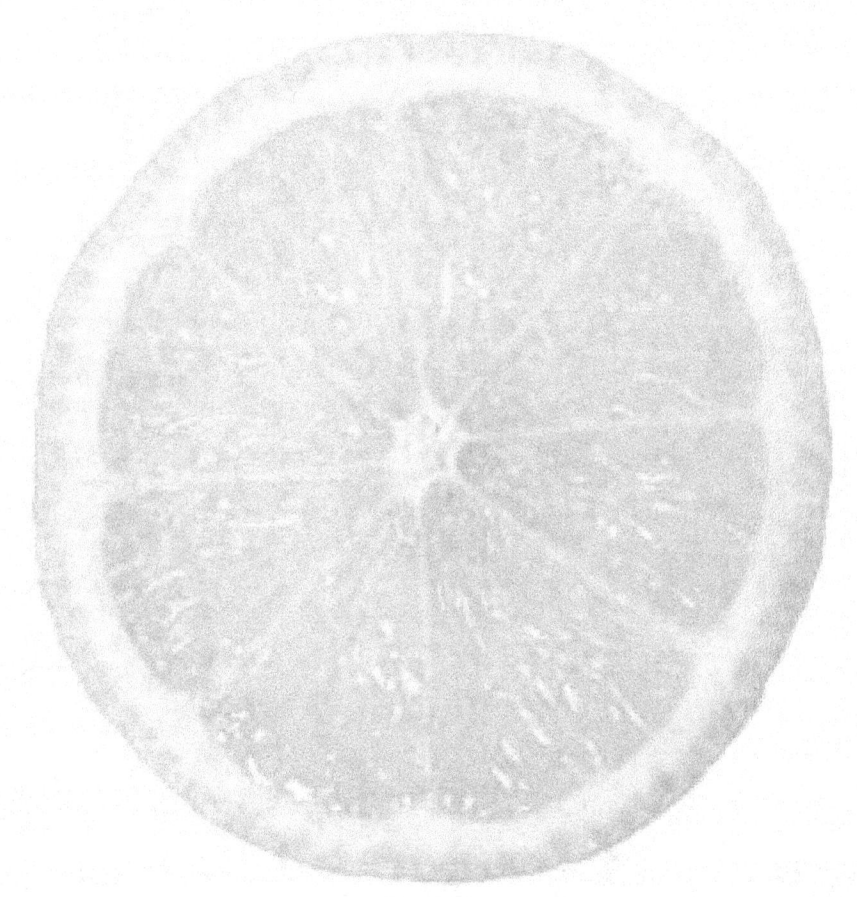

Squats, Squats, Squats!

People undergoing the 21 day sugar detox cleanse are not recommended to undertake any extreme workout plan; however you can always do squats. Press ups and squats are proven to lower your blood sugar level by 60% and that too by only doing them for 5 minutes. Plus doing squats helps to balance the sugar levels in your blood and this stability leads to lesser cravings.

The Psychological Effects: How To Best Cope With What You Might Be Feeling

If the title of this chapter is making you feel jittery and drawn from the idea of a 21 day withdrawal of sugar, then you are definitely the perfect candidate to go through the following. Remember everything that was ever a success started off seeming impossible but not with hesitation in any part from the person embarking on the decision.

And the fact that sugar has become the other half of a relationship for you is the perfect reason why you should give yourself 21 days to think about all the good things that are happening in your life without it.

Now the reason that I specifically mentioned the words : '....*how you might be feeling*' is due to the fact that what your mind might be going through is different for everyone as the effects of the detox are not identical either (we are talking about the invisible effects not the direct ones that you gain from a good detox).

When the body re-orients itself some people experience shakiness, mood swings, lethargy and sweatiness.

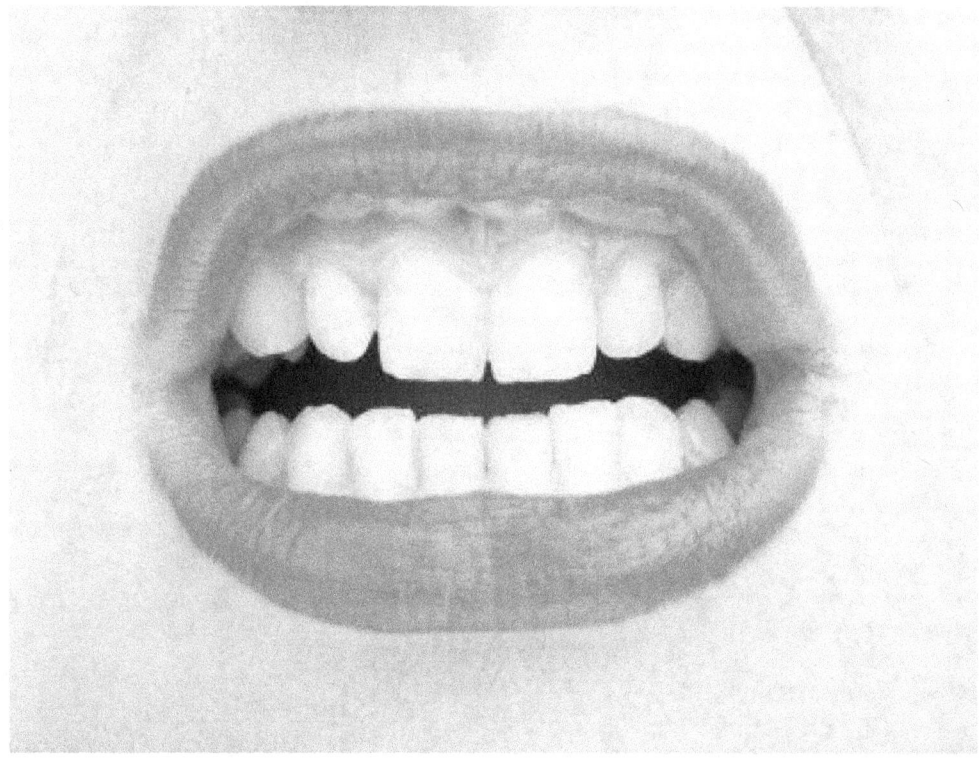

What Does Sugar Mean To Me?

According to experts all addictions pose physiological and physical triggers. Now when the body is not receiving food that it used to consume routinely, it will send out indicators in the form of cravings. Not just because you eat a lot of sugar but because pre historically our genes are used to consuming sweet food as organic food has a lot of nutrient density, the body will send out signals of sugar cravings even when it feels slightly dehydrated or hungry. So now you know what those cravings really mean.

A lot of psychologists believe that people are programmed from early childhood to associate sugar with reward, comfort and safety. This association is created by the common human rituals of offering lollipops for a job well done, having cake for birthdays and sweet treats during the holidays.

There is little left to the wonder about the relationship people have with sugar. The physical and the psychological triggers are not balanced in a person so it is your job to first figure out which is the more potent one for you.

What You Can Do:

1. Be Patient; Be Committed

Practice compassion. You are not your body's enemy. The cravings may seem cruel to ignore but remind yourself that these will eventually go away and not even turn back for a last glance at you. Remember, it is very important that you do not treat yourself as if you are punishing yourself for being addicted to sugar. Trust me where that train of thought is going will never benefit you. All you need to do is breathe (breathe deeply don't make that face, a little inhale and exhale does wonders). Tell yourself the truth; the punishment was when you were ingesting sugar; not now when you are freeing yourself from the addiction and undergoing the healing process. So be good to yourself!

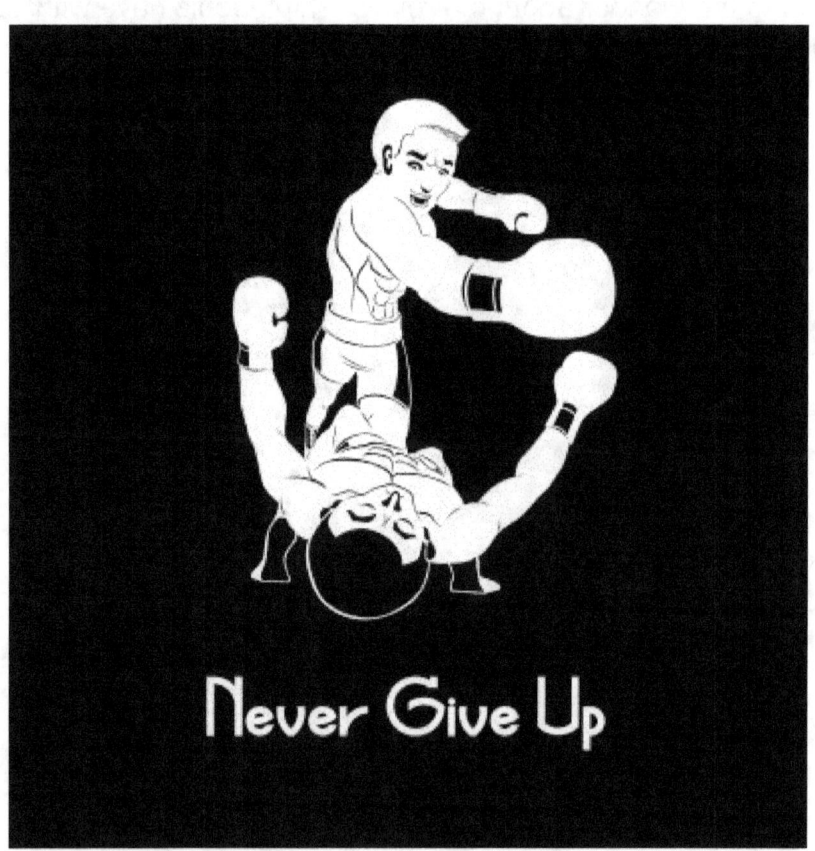

2. The Written Game Plan

Trust me, if you write down a well drafted plan for the entire detox period then dealing with the psychological triggers will be less exhausting and much easier to handle. For example when the triggers take effect you will deviate from the detox without even realizing it.

You can start doing this by first identifying what foods have sugar in them in your daily diet routines. Only after this will you be ready to draft a plan. Choose the start date of the 21 day detox and start from there on your calendar. Remember you will need to gather all the information you can that is going to help you out on your detox because you are fore-planning all that you are going to eat beforehand and now this plan is going to be the hard and fast rule for your daily menu for the next 21 days.

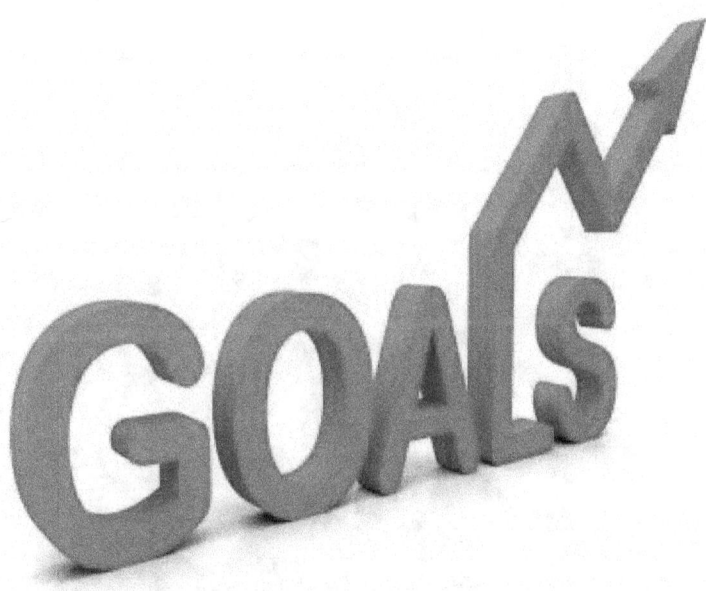

The first week into the detox regime you will not even remember what you planned out and the hassle of planning a sugar free meal again and again will be reduced. So basically your sugar detox now only requires the effort of you implementing it instead of contemplating it too.

3. Fill In The Spaces

Okay so you have eliminated the sugar from your diet, but now you are faced with a gaping hole in your dietary plan. This is a great opportunity for you to fill the portions up with things your body needs. First off, you need hydration and dense nutrition in place of sugar. This you will receive from foods rich in proteins and healthy fats.

Now when it comes to your psychological needs, start by adding substitutes for the sweet taste by eating root veggies and fruits. Your taste buds will soon adjust to the new natural sources. But remember never add sugar to the fruit serving. For instance people do add sugar to their fruit smoothies because the fruit does not taste sweet enough. Do not give in to the cravings like this; I repeat: DO NOT GIVE IN!

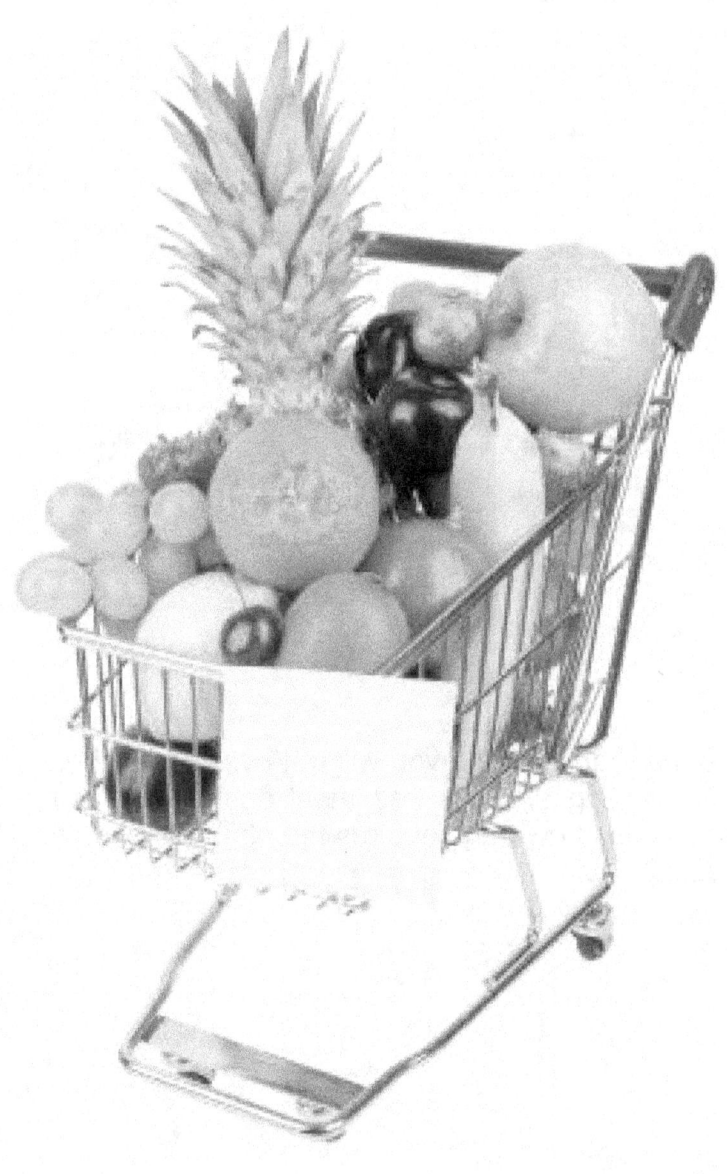

4. Buddy Up

It makes a huge difference to your motivation and mind set when you are among likeminded people. Find a sugar detox buddy to start the regime with you. You can share advice, suggestions and experiences and trust me if one does not give in to the cravings the other will keep going too.

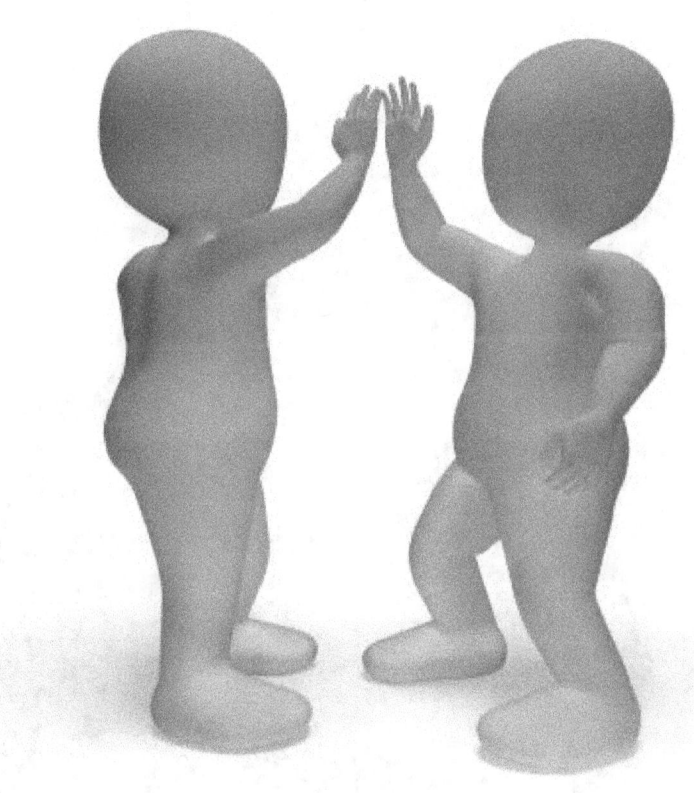

5. Let the World Know

Or you could simply go on about announcing what you are doing. Letting your friends and the people close to you know helps them be sensitive to your cravings and eventually know when they should binge on sugar when one out of the group is on a detox. When the sugar is out of sight it will be out of mind too.

I think preparing your mind for any such practices or regimes or a change of lifestyle is extremely important. For beginners even more so because if one can figure out this aspect, then the potential failure rate automatically reduces.

Having nutrition give you a hard time is nothing out of the ordinary. It is not just about going crazy over the withdrawal but according to experts, nutritional imbalances are a key factor in affecting your mental health (right next to impacting on your physical health).

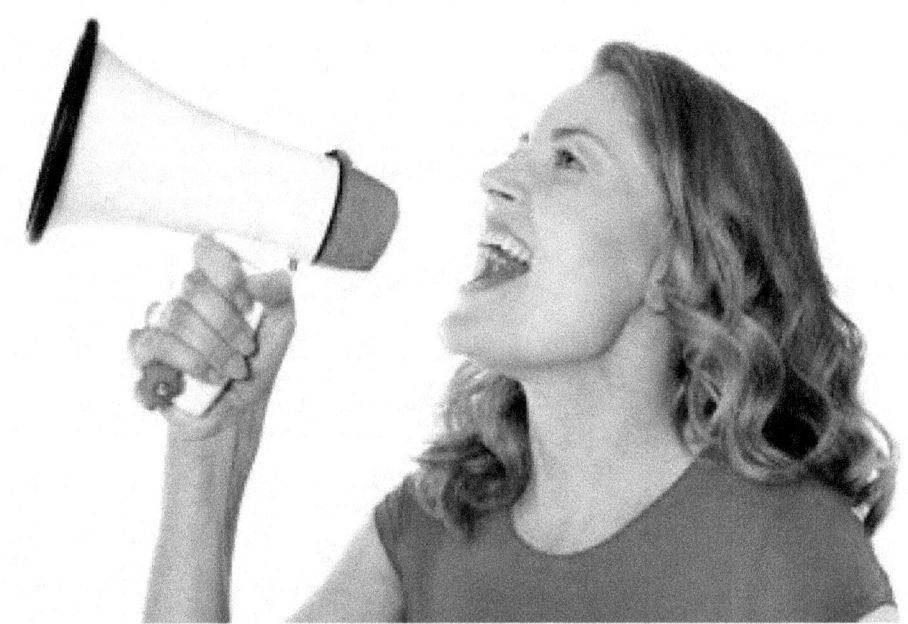

6. Spring Clean the Kitchen

Accompany a black bin bag to the kitchen and check all the labels of all your foods in the cabinets and the fridge. Drop anything that has sugar listed in its ingredients. Plus if the packed product has sugar listed as the first ingredient then it means that it is predominantly sugar inclusive. Everything that you throw in the bag must not be taken out and seen again. Just tie a knot and drop the bag in the garbage without a backward glance.

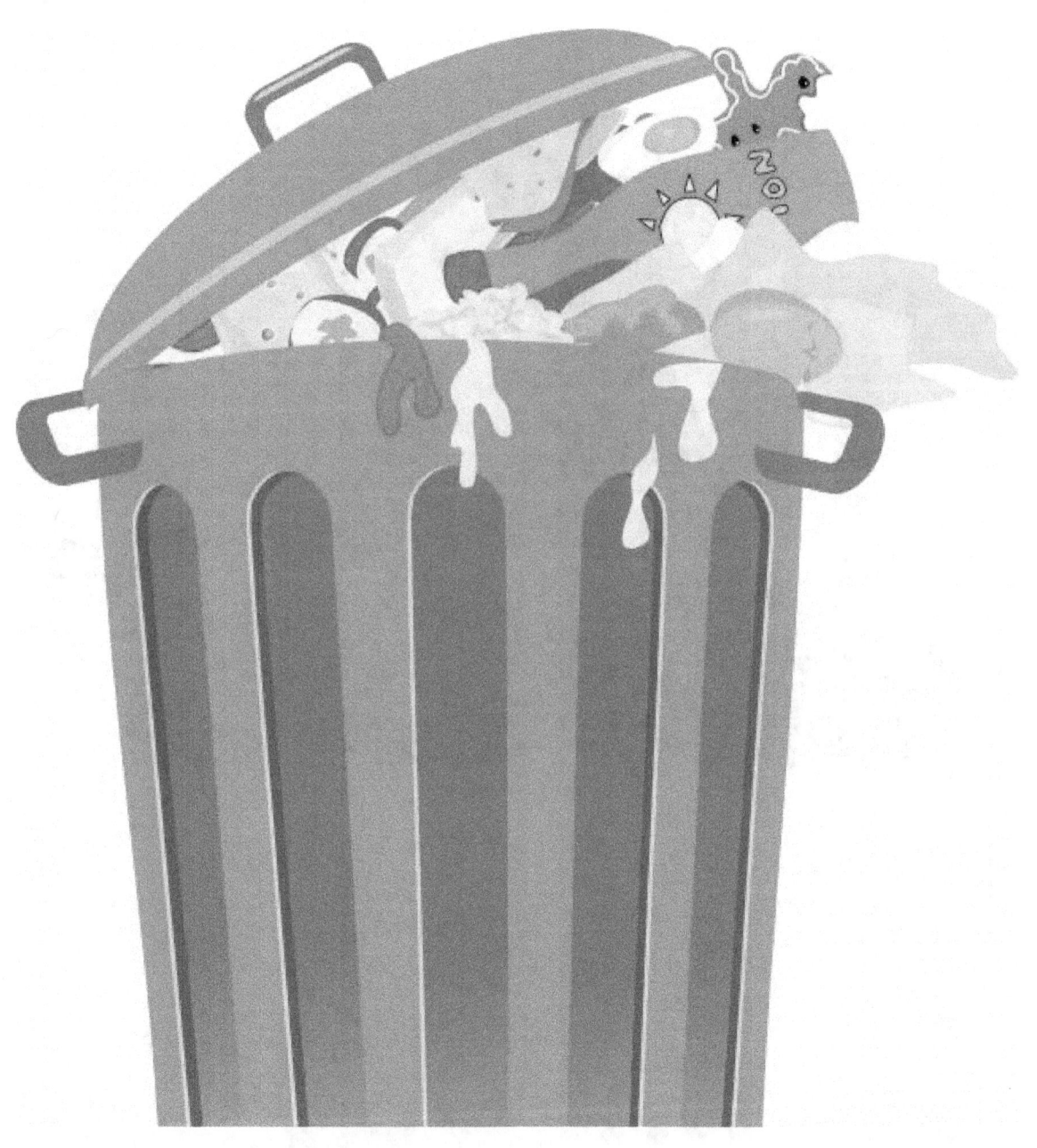

7. Meditation Helps

Meditating is simply awesome. It also aids in reducing mindless eating when you have nothing better to do and your mind is under the illusion that you are hungry. Meditating during a sugar detox works wonders. All you have to do is every day before you start a meal take a deep breath, take in the mouthwatering aroma of the food you are having and contemplate your appreciation for this food. Trust me your mind will wander miles from sugar, if thoughts of that are still lodged in the crevices of your brain.

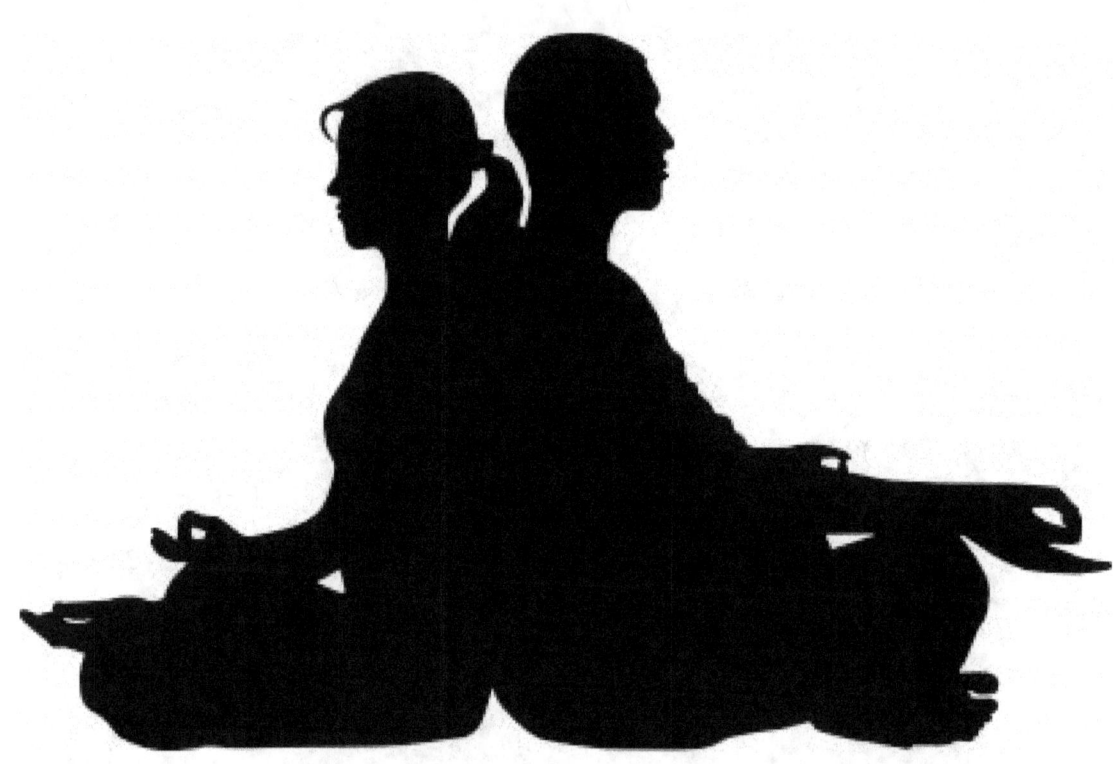

8. The Heart Wants What It Wants

There is a better solution than just bearing with the cravings. The best way to overcome something like that is if you take pleasure from other things around you; this will not only distract you but make your mind healthier. You will be strong against the sugar cravings and the desire for a sugar rush will reduce. You could start by a walk outside, a massage that you have been planning to get or some great music.

9. One Thought at A Time

The thing that will help you go through the entire 21 day detox is if you stop focusing on the big picture. I mean it is important that you are focused on your goal and the entire value of the 3 week detox. Focus on one step at a time. You have already drafted the entire plan all you need to do now is just master them. Bit by bit it will not look like as much of a burden to you and before you know it you would have breezed by the 21 days successfully.

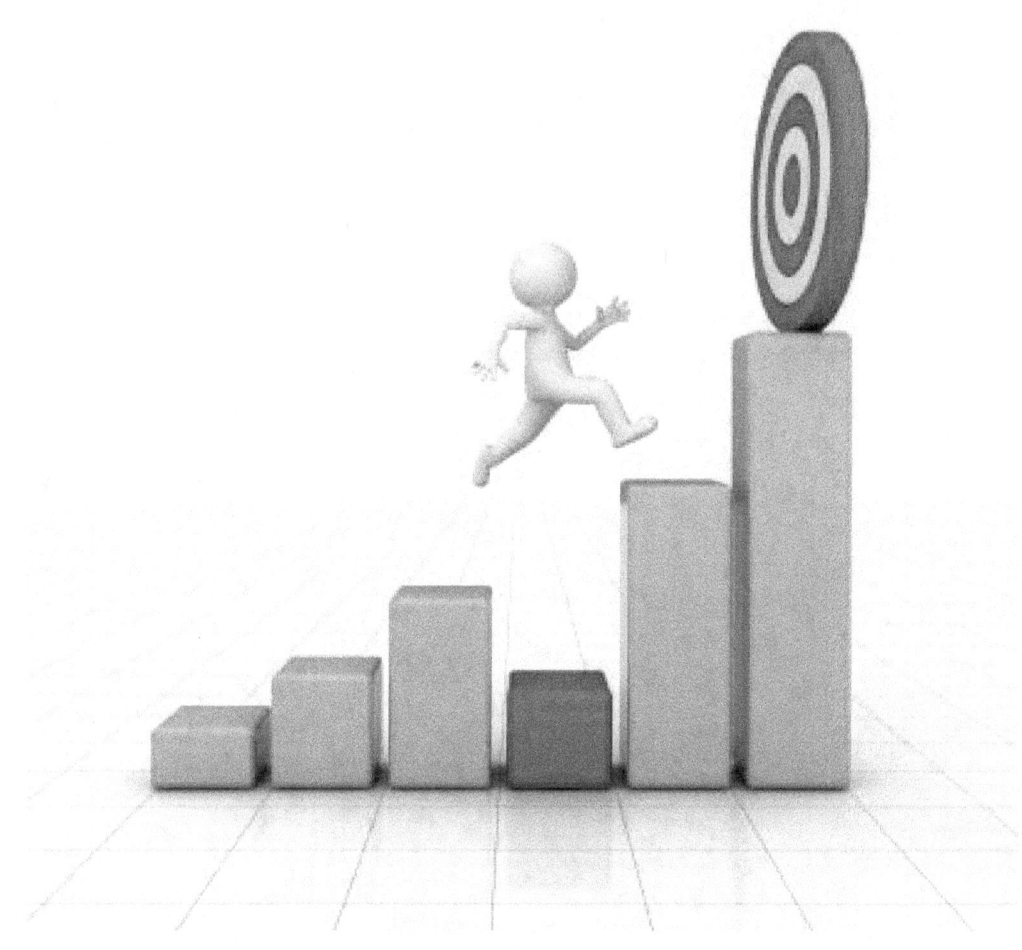

The Initial steps of the detox must not be mistaken for the baby steps. To stay on track for the following 21 days all you need to do is focus on the first few days. Make them pro sugar detox, for example turn your kitchen into the anti-sugar zone and spend the first few days on drafting sugar free recipes. When you really want change it becomes easier to achieve it.

www.ingramcontent.com/pod-product-compliance
Lightning Source LLC
Chambersburg PA
CBHW052016280526
45793CB00005B/1002